FATTY LIVER DIET

A Total Guide And Healthy Recipe To Help Lose Weight And Reverse Fatty Liver

SCOTT LARRY

Table of Contents

CHAPTER ONE 3
  INTRODUCTION 3
CHAPTER TWO 4
  TREATING FATTY LIVER WITH FOOD 4
CHAPTER THREE 12
  FOODS TO AVOID FOR A FATTY LIVER 12
CHAPTER FOUR 20
  FOODS TO CONSUME FOR A FATTY LIVER ... 20
THE END 24

CHAPTER ONE

INTRODUCTION

There are two major types of fatty liver ailment — alcohol-caused and nonalcoholic fatty liver ailment. Fatty liver sickness affects almost one-third of Yankee adults and is one of the main individuals to liver failure. Nonalcoholic fatty liver disorder is most generally recognized in people who are obese or sedentary and people who eat an extraordinarily processed weight-reduction plan.

CHAPTER TWO

TREATING FATTY LIVER WITH FOOD

One of the essential methods to deal with fatty liver disease, irrespective of kind, is with diet. Because the name suggests, fatty liver ailment way you have too much fats on your liver. In a healthful body, the liver enables to take away pollutants and produces bile, the digestive protein. Fatty liver sickness damages the liver and stops it from working as properly because it should.

In widespread, the weight-reduction plan for fatty liver disease consists of:

- Masses of end result and veggies

- Excessive-fiber vegetation like legumes and complete grains

- Very little brought sugar, salt, trans fat, subtle carbohydrates, and saturated fats

- No alcohol

A low-fat, reduced-calorie food plan let you lose weight and reduce the hazard of fatty liver ailment. Preferably, in case you're overweight, you'll intention to lose at the least 10percentt of your body weight.

Right here are some foods to also include to your healthy liver weight loss program:

1. Coffee to decrease bizarre liver enzymes.

Espresso drinkers with fatty liver disease have much less liver harm than individuals who don't drink this caffeinated beverage. Caffeine seems to decrease the quantity of unusual liver enzymes of people at risk for liver sicknesses.

2. Greens to prevent fats buildup

Broccoli is proven to assist prevent the buildup of fat in the liver in mice. Consuming more veggies, like spinach, Brussels sprouts, and kale, also can assist with preferred weight loss

3. Tofu to reduce fat buildup

A examine on rats observed that soy protein, that's contained in meals like tofu, may lessen fats buildup within the liver. Plus, tofu is low in fats and excessive in protein.

4. Fish for infection and fat stages
Fatty fish such as salmon,

sardines, tuna, and trout are excessive in omega-3 fatty acids. Omega-3 fatty acids can help enhance liver fats degrees and produce down irritation.

5. Oatmeal for energy

Carbohydrates from entire grains like oatmeal deliver your body energy. Their fiber content material additionally fills you up, which will let you keep your weight.

6. Walnuts to improve the liver

3 nuts are excessive in omega-3 fatty acids that human beings with fatty liver ailment who consume

walnuts have stepped forward liver feature tests.

7. Avocado to assist protect the liver

Avocados are high in healthy fats, and they incorporate chemical substances that would gradual liver damage. They're additionally rich in fiber, which could help with weight manipulate.

8. Milk and different low-fat dairy to defend from harm

Dairy is high in whey protein, which may additionally guard the liver from in addition harm.

9. Sunflower seeds for antioxidants

Those nutty-tasting seeds are excessive in diet E, an antioxidant which can protect the liver from further harm.

10. Olive oil for weight control

This healthful oil is excessive in omega-three fatty acids. It's healthier for cooking than margarine, butter, or shortening. Reveals that olive oil facilitates to decrease liver enzyme levels and control weight.

11. Garlic to help lessen body weight

This herb no longer handiest provides taste to food, however experimental studies also display that garlic powder dietary supplements may additionally assist reduce body weight and fats in people with fatty liver disease.

CHAPTER THREE

FOODS TO AVOID FOR A FATTY LIVER

There are absolutely meals you must keep away from or limit if you have fatty liver disorder. These ingredients usually make a contribution to weight benefit and increasing blood sugar.

• Alcohol. Alcohol is a major cause of fatty liver disease in addition to different liver illnesses.

Alcohol is the maximum common purpose of fatty liver ailment. Alcohol affects the liver, contributing to fatty liver ailment and different liver diseases, which includes cirrhosis.

A person with fatty liver disorder ought to lessen their intake of alcohol or eliminate it from their weight loss program altogether.

• Brought sugar. Stay away from sugary meals together with sweet, cookies, sodas, and fruit juices. High blood sugar will increase the quantity of fats buildup inside the liver. Introduced sugars make a contribution to excessive blood sugar tiers and might boom fat within the liver.

Producers often add sugar to sweet, ice cream, and sweetened beverages, along with soda and fruit drinks.

Brought sugars additionally feature in packaged meals, baked items, and even store-bought espresso and tea. Keeping off other sugars, including fructose and corn syrup, also can assist limit fats in the liver.

• Fried foods. These are excessive in fat and energy. Too much fried food is possibly to growth calorie intake and the hazard of weight benefit. Weight problems are a commonplace cause of fatty liver disorder.

Including more spices and herbs to a meal is an exceptional manner to taste ingredients without including salt. Humans also can typically bake or steam ingredients in place of frying them.

- Salt. Consuming too much salt can make your frame hold on to extra water. Restriction sodium to much less than 1,500 milligrams according to day.

- White bread, rice, and pasta. White generally way the flour is particularly processed, that could enhance your blood sugar greater than entire grains because of a lack of fiber.

- Red meat. Red meat and deli meats are high in saturated fat.

In addition to editing your diet, right here are some other ways of life modifications you can make to improve your liver health:

1. Get greater lively. Exercising, paired with food regimen, permit you to lose more weight and manipulate your liver disorder. Aim to get at least half-hour of cardio exercising on most days of the week.

2. Lower LDL cholesterol. Watch your saturated fats and sugar intake to assist hold your LDL cholesterol and triglyceride tiers under manipulate. If weight-reduction plan and exercise aren't enough to lower your cholesterol, ask your doctor about taking medication.

3. Control diabetes. Diabetes and fatty liver disorder often occur together. Eating regimen and exercising let you manage both situations. In case your blood sugar is still excessive, your medical doctor can prescribe medication to lower it.

4. Delicate grains. Processed and subtle grains are found in white bread, white pasta, and white rice. Manufacturers have removed the fiber from these fairly processed grains that can enhance blood sugar as the frame breaks them down.

A look at of a 73 adults with nonalcoholic fatty liver ailment discovered that folks who ate up fewer refined grains had a decrease hazard of metabolic syndrome — a collection of hazard factors that increase the probability of coronary heart ailment and stroke.

Humans can without problems update subtle grains with potatoes, legumes, or entire-wheat and complete-grain alternatives.

CHAPTER FOUR

FOODS TO CONSUME FOR A FATTY LIVER

A weight loss program for fatty liver ailment should encompass a huge form of foods.

Reducing calorie intake and ingesting high fiber, natural ingredients is a great starting point. Ingesting foods that incorporate complicated carbohydrates, fiber, and protein can offer sustained energy and sell satiety.

Foods that lessen infection or assist the frame repair its cells are equally important.

Some humans select to follow unique food regimen plans, such as a plant-primarily based weight loss plan or the Mediterranean diet. A dietitian can regularly assist someone create a custom designed diet plan this is right for their tastes, signs, and fitness reputation.

Further to these simple recommendations, some specific foods may be particularly helpful for humans with fatty liver sickness. These meals encompass:

Garlic

Garlic is a staple in lots of diets, and it may provide blessings for human beings with fatty liver disorder. Garlic powder dietary supplements appear to assist reduce body weight and fat in the ones who have fatty liver sickness.

Coffee

Drinking espresso is a morning ritual for plenty humans. However, it could offer advantages past a burst of electricity for people with fatty liver ailment.

Animal look at located that decaffeinated espresso reduced

liver harm and irritation in mice that ate a weight loss program containing high tiers of fats, fructose, and LDL cholesterol.

THE END

Printed in the USA
CPSIA information can be obtained
at www.ICGtesting.com
LVHW020418150424
777424LV00007B/649